THE ESSENTIAL HANDBOOK TO CARB CYCLING AND THE KETOGENIC DIET

How to make the changes needed to be successful with carb cycling and how it relates to the Keto Diet including Frequent Questions, Meal Plans, and Shopping Lists

BY

EVELYN CARMICHAEL

Evelyn Carmichael

FORWARD

Many of my readers have requested that I write an easy to understand Essential Handbook on the Ketogenic Diet. I have resisted thinking perhaps this diet was a fad but have become more and more convinced that it can be a useful tool and part of an overall lifestyle change. This diet has more preconceived negatives than most that I have covered, but as the research grows, the overwhelming consensus shows that used effectively this diet can not only reduce weight but reduce inflammation, lower blood sugars, reduce heart disease, and even lower bad cholesterol.

It's not an eat all the bacon I want to diet. Nor can one stuff themselves with the ever so popular fat bombs (peanut butter cups) they want. Used properly, it can be an effective way to get to your goal weight. Carb Cycling is a popular derivative of Ketogenic Diet. Having set times or days for low carb eating may fit better into your lifestyle or be used as a step down from the Keto Diet.

Evelyn Carmichael

TABLE OF CONTENTS

LEGAL NOTES

Copyright © 2019 Evelyn Carmichael

All rights reserved.

INTRODUCTION

If you are considering going on a diet you may have heard of the very popular Ketogenic diet and the derivative Carb Cycling Diet. This diet has found worldwide acclaim thanks to its ability to help people lose weight and keep it off for good. While there are a lot of other diets out there it seems that the Ketogenic diet is a highly effective one that continues to make headlines even today.

Carb Cycling is a variation that you will learn about that take components of the Keto Diet and is modified to fit your lifestyle. This handbook will explain what Keto and Carb Cycling is and how to understand the world of macronutrients so you can successfully count carbs. If you're serious about losing weight and you want a sustainable diet change, the Ketogenic diet could be successful for you.

People who are ultimately successful on the Keto diet has a good understanding of macronutrients. This is discussed a lot in this book, but basically it is a grasp on the building blocks of the food you eat and how it effects your body. Keeping track of your net carbs is vital to success and this book will teach you how to do so at home and when you go out to eat. While some diets are about calorie counting, this is more of an accounting of what the food is made of that you are consuming.

Once you understand the Keto diet, you may want to modify this diet plan to do carb cycling. This handbook will explain what carb cycling is and you will be able to determine which method best fits your lifestyle.

If you are diabetic, pregnant, breastfeeding or you have had your gallbladder removed you will need to make some adjustments that are discussed in this book. This Essential Handbook will tell you how to stick to the Ketogenic diet while ensuring your body gets the nutrients it always needs . As with any type of diet, make sure you consult with your physician before starting.

Evelyn Carmichael

CHAPTER 1. HOW DOES THE KETOGENIC DIET WORK?

The Ketogenic Diet has been proven to help you lose weight. This diet works by ensuring you limit your intake of carbohydrates so that your body begins to burn fat as opposed to sugar. When your body burns energy it firstly begins to burn any blood sugar (Carbohydrates) that you've eaten. As soon as the sugar has been burned your body will begin to burn stored fat (ketone bodies). This is called ketosis.

When you start eating according to the 'Rules' of the Ketogenic Diet you will start to eat fewer carbohydrates. This means that your body will burn fewer sugars simply because you haven't consumed as many and will, therefore, burn more fat. It is this aspect of the diet that ensures you're are much more likely to lose weight. In other words, you will burn more fat than you'll consume, which is ideal for weight loss.

How long does it take for the body to switch from using blood sugar to ketone bodies?

After just 2-4 days on the Keto Diet, your body will start to make big changes. It will begin to go into ketosis and start using stored fat for energy. For most individuals, this is accomplished by eating 20 to 50 grams of carbohydrates a day.

MACRONUTRIENTS

Macronutrients are the building blocks of your diet and consist of protein, carbohydrates, and fats. Getting your macronutrient ratio right is essential as macronutrients form the base of your diet. Getting your macronutrients right is essential as doing so will help you to lose weight.

MACRONUTRIENTS

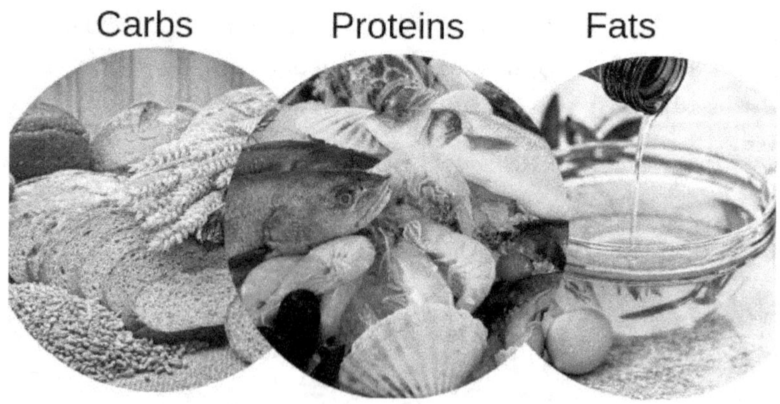

You should ideally get no more than ten percent of your calories from carbohydrates. No more than thirty percent of your calories from protein and no more than 60 percent of your calories from fat. It is essential that you work out where all your calories come from. When you can get the macronutrient ration right you will start to lose weight. This is because the macronutrients will come from many different sources rather than meals that are full of fat and sugar.

HOW DO I KNOW IF I AM IN KETOSIS?

The chart below shows some of the signs of being in ketosis. While some signs are positive, such as losing weight, there are some side effects, such as ketone breath (fruity smelling) that may be found. Also, while the chart shows some more obvious signs, a blood test is the most definitive measure to show ketones in your blood. Blood test results will show .5-3 millimoles of blood ketones per liter. There are at home breath and urine kits available as well.

PROOF?

Due to the popularity of the Ketogenic Diet, there have been many studies examining the effect of the Ketogenic Diet and its effect on weight loss. One of the early studies in 2004 looked at the long- time effects of the diet (24 weeks) and found that not only did Body Mass Index BMI) decrease significantly but bad cholesterol levels (LDL) went down and good cholesterol (HDL) levels went up. Triglyceride levels also decreased significantly.   Furthermore, a 2017 study looked at the Ketogenic Diet in Endocrine Disorders and found that there is clinical evidence to support the use of KD in diabetes, obesity, and endocrine disorders.

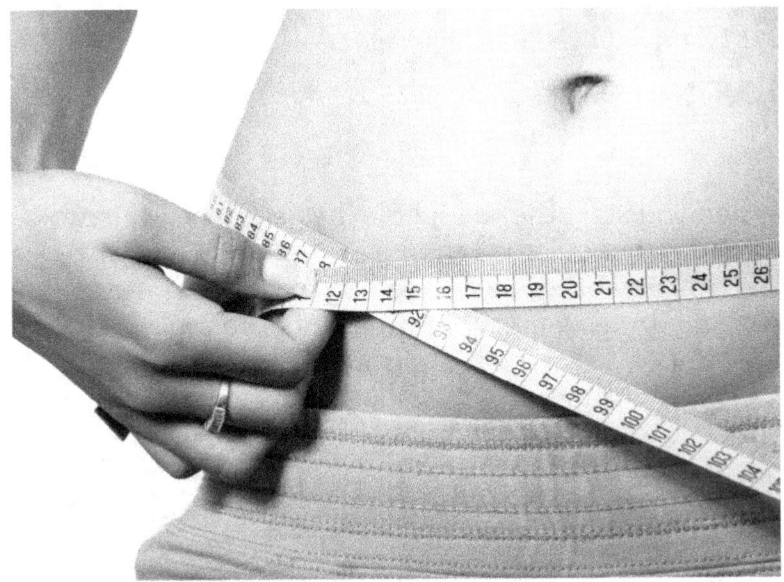

Signs of Ketosis

Decreased Appetite
Weight Loss
Ketosis Breath
Short-Term Fatigue
Decrease in Productiveness
High Energy
Digestive Issues
Muscle Cramps
Headaches
Increased Focus

BECOMING IN TUNE WITH WHAT YOU ARE EATING

When you start the Ketogenic diet, you need to pay attention to your food intake just as you would if you were on any other diet. Keeping track of calories, carbohydrates, and sugar intake of each food, especially while you are trying to reach ketosis is vitally important to not sabotage your diet. While your intake of carbohydrates will be low, there is every chance that you could still put weight on. Therefore, it's important that you keep an eye on the calories you consume.

THE BENEFITS OF THE KETOGENIC DIET

The Ketogenic Diet is quite an easy diet to stick to. This is because the diet involves you eating a lot of tasty foods and it helps you lose weight. The meals that you will be enjoying as part of the Ketogenic diet is likely to widen the variety of foods you eat. It will, therefore, help your body get more of the nutrients it needs. The more nutrients your body gets, the healthier you will be.

It may take you up to 2 months to get used to this diet. During the first 8 weeks, it's likely that you'll eat some foods that contain a lot more carbohydrates than you imagine. Do not worry about this. You can start from scratch again then next time you eat something. Making a few mistakes is normal don't beat yourself up about it, it happens to us all.

- It Burns Fat

The Ketogenic diet is great at helping you to burn fat. When you partake in this diet your body goes into Ketosis. Ketosis occurs when you burn more sugars/carbohydrates than you eat. If you consume fewer carbohydrates your body will start to burn more fat, and this results in weight loss.

We consider fat to be quite unhealthy, this is because it can out a bit of a strain on our vital organs. When you lose weight and burn the fat away you will start to put less strain on your vital organs. Weight loss is often accompanied by better self-estecm.

- It's Good for your Sugar Levels

The Ketogenic can be good at helping to lower your sugar levels. Those with diabetes or those are likely to develop this condition may find that the Ketogenic diet stabilizes their sugar level. You should always keep an eye on your sugar level if you have diabetes or you think you may develop it. The Ketogenic diet is no substitute for the care provided by your doctor.

OTHER BENEFITS OF THE KETOGENIC DIET

The other benefits of the Ketogenic diet include:

- ✓ More energy over throughout the day with your energy levels less likely to dip
- ✓ Less heartburn and indigestion
- ✓ Fewer sugar cravings
- ✓ A reduction in inflammation
- ✓ A less irritable bowel
- ✓ An improved digestive system
- ✓ A lowered risk of heart disease

I thought eating a lot of meat increased cholesterol?

When you tell someone you are on the Keto Diet, you may inevitably hear something to the effect of "I could never do that diet, my cholesterol would be through the roof eating all that meat." When eating true to the Keto Diet though, the exact opposite has shown to occur. Compared to a low-fat,

Evelyn Carmichael

Chapter 2. Seriously, What Can I Eat and More Importantly, Not Eat?

One of the great things about the Ketogenic diet is that it's less restrictive than many other diets. When you restrict your intake, you're more likely to have difficulties sticking to the diet. What's more, is you're likely to eat something that is on your diets 'Forbidden' list. A lot of people tend to miss the foods they enjoy when they're on a diet, but this is not the case with the Ketogenic Diet. In fact, this particular diet insists that you consume foods that leave you satisfied.

What this means is you are more likely to stick with the Ketogenic Diet than you are any type of diet. You are therefore more likely to stick with it and reach your weight goals and feel better about your body, and that is never a bad thing.

While you may not be able to eat as much bread or as many fries as you may wish to, the good news is there are a lot of other foods you can eat. Filling, nutritious and satisfying, these foods will leave you feeling as though you're not really on a diet after all.

NET VS TOTAL CARBS

The goal to get into ketosis is to stay under 20 to 50 grams of net carbohydrates per day. To pinpoint your exact range of carbs and you will need to pay attention to your body to see the signs that you are in ketosis. If after a few days you don't see any of the signs drop your carbohydrate intake.

Make sure when you are looking at your carbohydrate intake you are looking at the net carbs vs. total carbohydrates. To do this, you need to make sure you know how to read a nutritional label. While some labels will have net carbs listed, many do not. An easy way to figure out the net carbs is to take the total carbohydrates and subtract the amount of fiber to get the actual net carb amount.

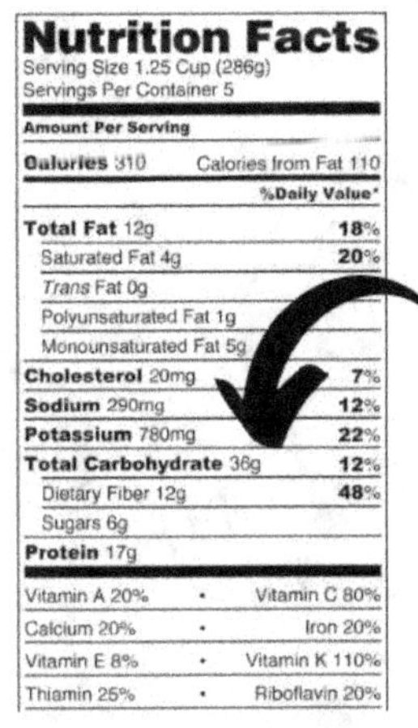

Find Net Carb Value

Total Carb= 36

Subtract Fiber - 12

Net Carb Value= 24

Note: If the label has more than 5 added alcohol sugar, you can subtract half the amount. For example, if the total carbs were 30g with 0 grams of fiber, and there are 12g of alcohol sugars, the total number of net carbs would be 24grams.

HEALTHY LOW CARB FOOD CHOICES

Take a look at the following charts to see a sampling of healthy keto foods. These are foods that are high in protein, fiber, and good for you oils/fats. Gravitate towards grass fed or organic meat varieties and low to no processed foods.

Evelyn Carmichael

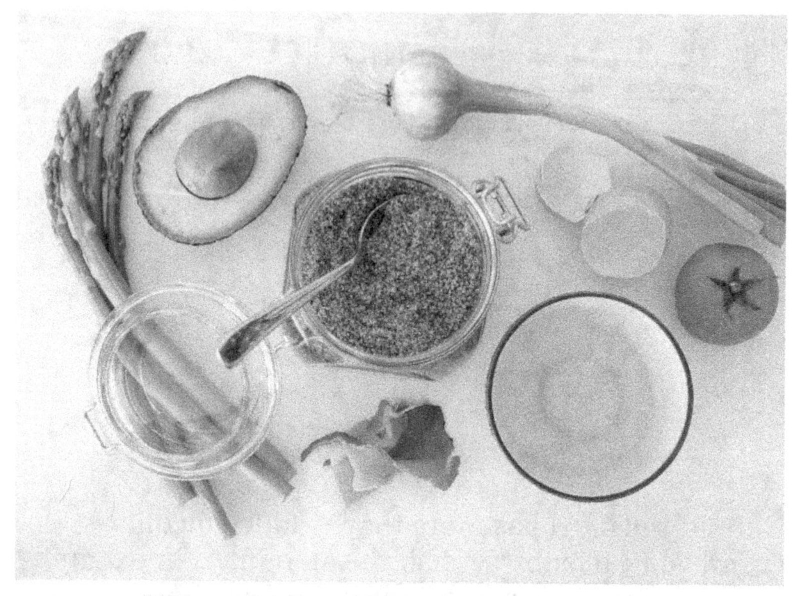

Healthy Keto Foods

Eggs
Avocado
Fish and Shellfish
Low Carb Vegetables
Olive and Coconut Oil
Grass Fed Meat
Cheese
Berries

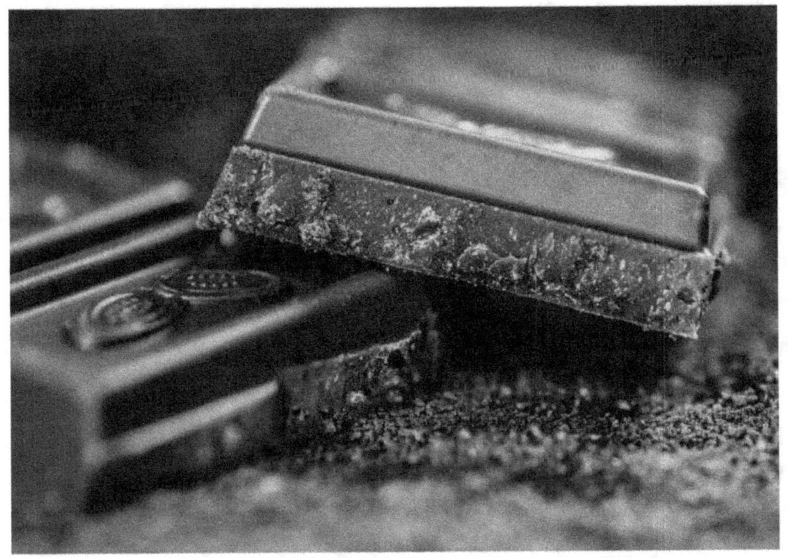

Healthy Keto Snacks

Dark Chocolate

Cherry Tomatoes

Guacomole

Nuts and Seeds

Peanut Butter Cups

String Cheese

Deviled Eggs

Pork Rinds

Beef Jerky

Hummus

Evelyn Carmichael

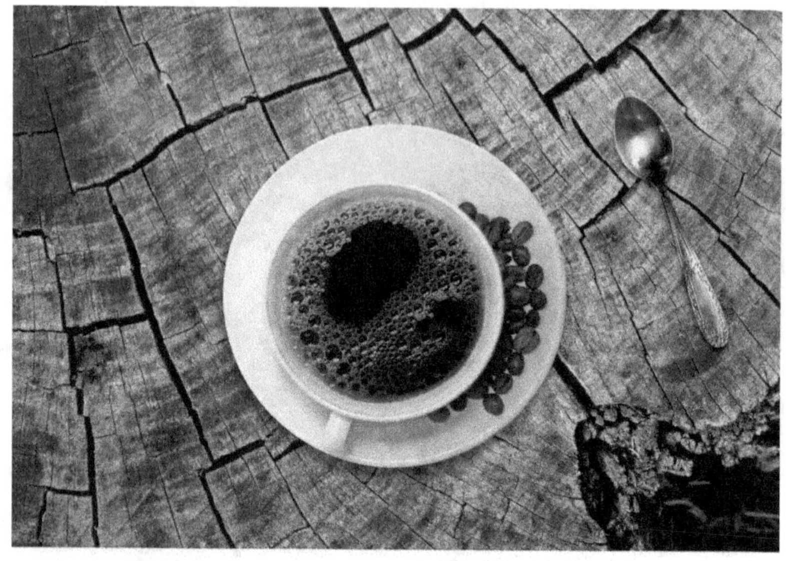

Healthy Keto Drinks

Water

Coffee

Tea-unsweetened

Sparkling water

Broths

Alcohol in moderation: Wine

Hard Spirts (pair only with soda water)

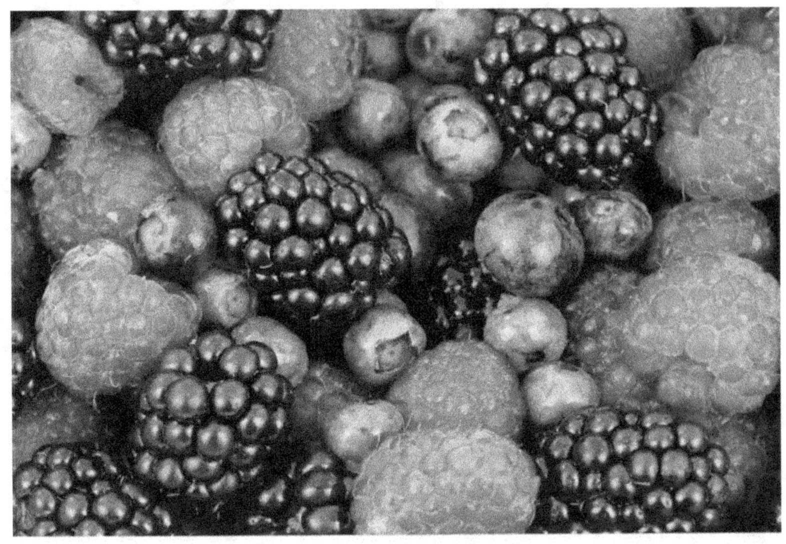

Fruit

Fruit	Net Carbs	Serving
Blackberries	4	1/2 cup
Raspberries	3	1/2 cup
Blueberries	9	1/2 cup
Strawberries	5	5 med. sized
Banana	21	1 medium
Plum	7	1 medium
Apple	12	1 small
Cherries	8	1/2 cup
Cantaloupe	11	1 cup

WHAT FOODS SHOULD I STAY AWAY FROM?

While some people think that the Ketogenic Diet is one of the lesser restrictive diets, you do need to be careful to watch your carbohydrate as well as the amount of sugars that you consume daily. Ideally, you should avoid any food that contains a lot of carbohydrates, meat that has been processed or factory farmed, and any highly processed foods.

You should also try to stay away from:

- Milk – Milk is high in naturally occurring sugars and it can be hard for your body to digest. This is because aside from breast milk, we were not made to consume milk. You may, therefore, wish to drink a milk substitute such as soy, almond or coconut milk.

- Artificial sweeteners – Many sweeteners contain chemicals that make your brain tell your body that you're hungry. Artificial sweeteners can often be found in diet sodas, so you may want to avoid these.

- Alcohol – If you want to be successful at losing weight, you need to stay away from certain types of alcohol. This is because every alcoholic drink contains sugars, sometimes more than you would think. The sugars found in alcohol vary considerably. In general, beer and any alcohol mixed with anything but soda water is high in carbs and or sugar. Take for example beer. It contains an average whopping 13 carbs, which is a good chunk of your daily allowance for one beer! Alternatively, dry white and most red wines have 2 grams of sugar. What you add to the drink is often more damaging than the drink itself. Take a gin and tonic. At 14 grams of sugar, tonic water is full of sugars that will sabotage your diet. Switching to soda water, the sugars drop to zero.

- Foods that contain no carbohydrates – Food that contains no carbohydrates may also be advertised as containing very little fats. However, foods such as these are likely to have a lot of additives in them, along with artificial sweeteners. Pay close attention to the nutrition label on any processed foods advertised to be carb free.

- Refined fats and oils – Margarine, corn oil, sunflower oil, and canola oil are full of fats that are not good for you. Better alternatives are coconut oil, avocado oil, olive oil, ghee, and stevia.

Evelyn Carmichael

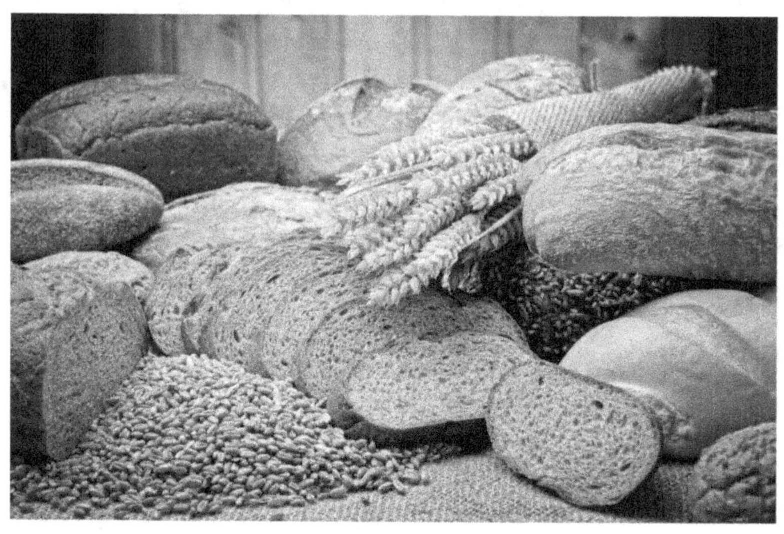

Foods to Avoid

Bread

Sugary Drinks

Potatoes

Pasta

Beans

Rice

Beer

Candy

Pastries/Donuts/Cake/Pie

Starchy Fruit (non-berry)

I'M CONFUSED, IS DAIRY GOOD OR BAD?

The short answer is both. Basically, the full fat dairy is good to eat as it has fatty acids (linoleic acid) that aid in fat loss. Butters, creams, and full fat cheeses fit the bill. Lower fat dairy such as skim milk, yogurts (exception being plain Greek yogurt), margarine, and low-fat dairy varieties do not have the acids needed and are higher in carbs and sugar.

SERIOUSLY, NO BEER AND MARGARITAS?

In general, no. However, there are some alternative beers and even sweet drinks like margaritas that are "skinny" style containing far less carbs and sugars. While this is ok for a once in a while cheat, remember that having artificial sweeteners is also not the best idea as it tricks your body into wanting more sugar.

Evelyn Carmichael

CHAPTER 3. WHAT IS CARB CYCLING?

You may have heard the term "Carb Cycling". This is where you have certain days of the week you eat foods that are higher in carbohydrates than other days. Carb cycling is a modified version of the Keto diet and is often used for when people have reached their goal weight and want to maintain their weight. Increasingly in popularity, some individuals are using carb cycling as a modified Keto Diet from the start.

Advantages of carb cycling:
- ✓ Higher carb days boost insulin levels to build and maintain muscle tissue
- ✓ Keeps your metabolism high
- ✓ Food variety is expanded

Carb cycling usually falls into two categories.

1) Exercise based. On the days you exercise you eat more carbs than on days you don't. So, if you go to the gym 4 days a week, those days

you eat a larger amount of carbs. The other 3, you stick to a very low carb meal plan.

2) Regimented Days. You have certain days of the week you eat low carb, the other days you eat don't eat low carb. Some people find the weekends harder to stick to a low carb diet and want the flexibility to eat more carbs. Eating low carb Monday through Friday may be easier when you have your set work routine and then you can ease some more carbs back in your diet on the weekend.

Another method is every other day you switch between a low and higher carb day.

It's important to make sure that with carb cycling you are not overdoing the carbs on the off days. You want to reload your carb stores but not overload them so that your body cannot get back into ketosis. If you are doing a modified ketogenic plan and want to get back into ketosis, you need to make sure your higher carb days are not too high so that you can easily get back into ketosis. A good rule of thumb is that higher carb days are no more than 30% higher than your lower carb days.

Carb Cycling is also sometimes referred to as a diet plan on its own, without going back into ketosis. Compliance may be the biggest factor of success with this diet. For a lot of individuals, having one cheat meal or day leads to many others. For those that are heavy exercise users, carb cycling has its benefits of increasing energy and reducing muscle fatigue. For those that are committed to their diet plan, knowing there is a "reward" day helps keep some on track. Finally, carb cycling done right can also assist with keeping your metabolism higher. Similar to varying your work outs, carb cycling can keep your body's metabolism from slowing down too much.

ALLOWING FOR A HIGHER CARB DAY

One of the more popular tips for success is allowing for one day a week of increased carb intake to 60 to 80 grams of carbs. Make sure that the increase in carbs is refined and not processed carbs. Ideally, this would be adding in some extra fruit or a starchy vegetable such as a sweet potato or tubular root veggie. Stay away from sweets such as candy, cookies, cake, or any type of pastry.

Some individuals find success with following the Keto Diet fairly strictly but allowing for a higher carb day per week. This is similar to combing a variant of carb cycling and the Keto diet into a happy medium that a lot of individuals can follow.

CHAPTER 4. HOW DO I EAT OUT, SHOP, AND MEAL PLAN?

The truth is, eating out has never been easier. Many restaurants now include the nutritional count either on their menu or on a supplemental menu they have available. When in doubt, stay away from carbs and sauces. Opt for a lettuce wrap vs a bun and always stick with an oil-based vinaigrette for a salad dressing. Don't want to skip dessert when everyone at the table is partaking? Ask the server to bring you some berries with real whipped cream on top- or better yet- hold the berries and indulge in some yummy whipped cream.

At the grocery store, have in mind your staples and pre-plan your meals before going in. Below is a sample 7-day meal plan. Make sure you are eating low carb foods and switch things up to keep your diet interesting.

	Breakfast	**Lunch**	**Dinner**
Sunday	Ham and Cheese Omelet	Grilled Salmon Burger on lettuce "bun", Avocado salsa	Grilled Lamb Chops with Balsamic Reduction, Asparagus, Salad
Monday	Protein Smoothie	Tuna Avocado Cups	Chicken Sir Fry
Tuesday	Cauliflower hash browns, egg	Chopped Salad	Blue Cheese and Mushroom Burger wrapped in Kale leaves, Garlic Soy

			Green Beans
Wednesday	Spinach Scrambled Eggs	Meatball with Zoodles (zucchini noodles)	Lemon Pepper Salmon, asparagus with hollandaise
Thursday	2 eggs over medium with 2 strips bacon	Grilled garlic shrimp with cauliflower rice bowl	Grilled Chicken Sausage with Peppers, Roasted Garlic Cauliflower
Friday	Protein Smoothie		Chicken Lettuce Cups
Saturday	Egg Muffin Cups	Grilled Chicken	6oz Steak, Cheesy

		Tender Salad	Broccoli, Sautéed Mushrooms

SHOPPING LIST

<u>Dairy</u>

- o Butter
- o Greek Yogurt- plain
- o Full fat String Cheese
- o Cottage Cheese
- o Cheese Cubes
- o Shredded Cheese
- o Eggs
- o Creamer- full fat
- o Butter (full fat)

<u>Vegetables/Fruits</u>

- o Avocados
- o Strawberries
- o Blackberries
- o Raspberries
- o Plums
- o Broccoli
- o Kale
- o Romaine
- o Broccoli
- o Cauliflower
- o Green Beans
- o Spinach
- o Cabbage
- o Edamame

<u>Meat/Seafood</u>

- o Grass fed ground beef
- o Chicken breasts
- o Salmon
- o Shrimp
- o Tilapia

- Bacon (nitrate free)
- Lamb chops
- Lean grass-fed steak

<u>Staples</u>

- Peanut butter
- Macadamia Nuts
- Pine Nuts
- Pecans
- Almonds
- Peanuts
- Sunflower seeds
- Unsweetened Tea
- Sparkling Water
- Coffee
- Olive Oil
- Coconut Oil
- Balsamic Vinegar
- Apple Cider Vinegar
- Mustard
- Mayonnaise
- Hot Sauce
- Soy Sauce
- Full fat salad dressings
- Canned salmon or tuna
- Coconut or Almond Flour

<u>Frozen Aisle</u>

- Cauliflower Rice
- Smoothie Boosts (Acai Power Greens)

- o Zoodles (Zucchini Spirals)
- o Veggies
- o Meatballs

- o Cauliflower Frozen pizza crust

Evelyn Carmichael

CHAPTER 5. HOW LONG CAN I DO THE KETO DIET?

Nutritional experts vary greatly on this. There are generally four different routes to take for long term planning. Some believe that being in ketosis should be relatively short term to help you get to a healthy weight. Once at that weight, one can introduce a balanced diet of carbs back in to their daily diet. Some people supplement this with intermittent fasting or going back on keto for a short period of time if they find they are gaining weight.

Others believe that some bodies function better by eating low carbs. After reaching your goal weight, one can slowly add their carb intake to 10-20 grams of additional carbs per day. For those that are borderline diabetic or have issues with their blood glucose or triglyceride levels, this may be an ideal way to reduce carbs/ sugars in their diet but adding some flexibility to enjoy a low to moderate amount of carbs.

Carb cycling is becoming a popular option as well, discussed later in this chapter.

Others believe that you can remain in ketosis for longer periods of time. For muscle building, one could increase caloric and protein intake while still following the basic keto diet. This coupled with an exercise program will keep the fat off while building muscle.

You may have heard of maintenance Keto. This is when you have reached your goal weight but are concerned that if you add the carbs back in to your diet, the weight will come back on too. Some individuals prefer to stay on this diet plan for long term. At your goal weight, you can stay in ketosis while increasing your caloric intake as to not lose more weight. Making sure not to add any additional carbs, you can raise your calories with lean proteins and fats.

Others switch to a modified carb cycling where they have one to three days of higher carb days, but generally stick to the Keto Diet.

Regardless of the long-term plan you choose, make sure you have a discussion with your doctor to see what is right for your specific medical needs.

SAFELY COMING OUT OF KETOSIS

Once you have reached your goal weight, coming out of ketosis and resuming a more balanced diet of carbs should be something you put some thought in to. Eating smaller, more refined carbs will be easier for your body to tolerate versus heavily processed carbs such as pies, cupcakes, and the like. For the first couple of weeks, try introducing carbs rich in protein and fiber such as beans and rice in to one meal per day. See how your body responds before adding unprocessed carbs. You don't want your blood sugar to spike and then crash after eating carbs or any of the GI (think constipation or diarrhea) that may accompany introducing carbs back in to your diet.

Evelyn Carmichael

CHAPTER 6. HINTS AND TIPS

Here are a few hints and tips to help ensure a success with a Ketogenic lifestyle.

ALL ABOUT THE SAUCE

A common pitfall in your daily carb intake is not watching the sauce. If you are eating a chicken breast smothered in teriyaki sauce, you could be sabotaging your net carb allowance. At 5.7 net carbs per two tablespoons, a sauce laden dish can easily add up. Going light on the sauce or switching with soy sauce at .9 net carbs per two tablespoons will be a better alternative. Below is a chart of common condiments/ sauces.

Evelyn Carmichael

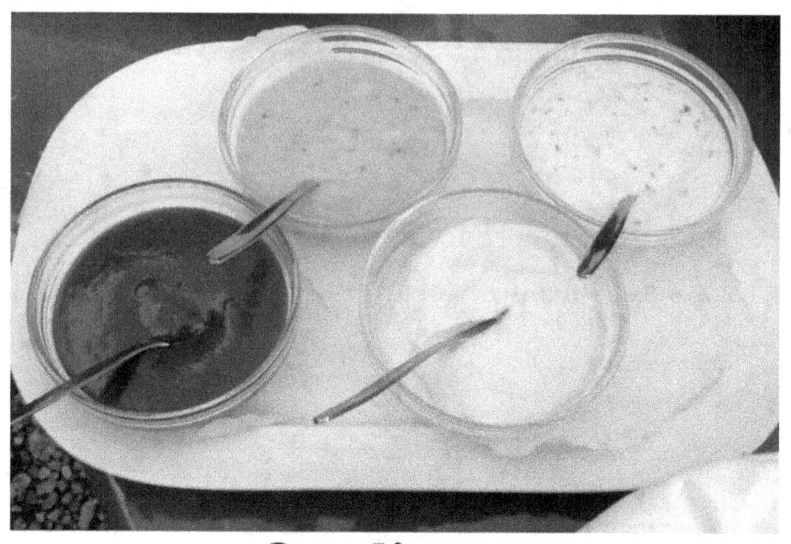

Condiments

Item	Net Carbs	Serving
Ketchup	4	1 TBS
Dijon Mustard	.5	1 Tsp
Mayonaise	.1	1 tsp
Soy Sauce	.9	1 TBS
Barbeque Sauce	3.6	2 TBS
Marinara Sauce	4.1	1/4 cup
Pesto Sauce	.6	1 TBS
Balsamic Vinegar	2.3	1 TBS
Teriyaki Sauce	5.7	2TBS
Tarter Sauce	1.1	2 TBS
Honey	5.8	1 Tsp

EATING TOO MUCH

If your goal of the Ketogenic Diet is to get down to a healthy weight, then you must watch how much you are eating per day. You will need to still monitor total caloric intake. While the food you are eating is higher in fat to get into ketosis, this is not an "all the bacon you can eat" diet. Sensible portions will leave you satisfied without overeating.

WHAT ARE SOME OF THE NEGATIVES I'VE HEARD ABOUT?

There have been some rumors about the Ketogenic and some less than desirable side effects. Knowing these potential side effects can help you combat them before they even begin.

Keto Flu

When you are eating very few carbs, your body is forced to use ketones instead of glucose (carbs) for energy. For some people, this causes symptoms that can be equated as if you are withdrawing from caffeine such as headaches while others may develop some flu like symptoms as their body adjusts to lower carb eating.

This can include:
- nausea
- vomiting
- constipation
- diarrhea
- muscle cramps/soreness
- irritability
- weakness/dizziness

These symptoms generally do not last longer than a week and can be combatted with staying hydrated, eating the maximum carbs, replacing electrolytes, and avoiding heavy exercise.

Keto Breath

When your body enters ketosis, you produce ketones. One of these ketones, acetone (an ingredient found in nail polish remover), is responsible for this not so great smell. This is an indicator that your keto diet is working and will go away as your body gets used to the low carb eating. To quicken this process, stay hydrated to excrete the ketones from your body.

Vaginal Odor

Along with Keto Breath, there have been reports of some women noticing different smells in their vaginal area. When you change your diet, your entire pH balance changes which can cause different smells. What you want to make sure of is that the smell is not a sign of a yeast infection. Your doctor can rule that out. Taking a probiotic to make sure your gut is producing good bacteria will also assist in your overall pH balance.

Muscle Loss

While there are a few rumors that the Ketogenic diet can result in muscle loss, it's unlikely that you will lose any muscle. This diet works by helping to lose weight as opposed to fat. If you continue to exercise as you normally would you will keep your muscles, but you will burn off more fat. So, for example, your arms may not be as round as they once were, but they will still have the same amount of muscle.

WHAT IS THE END RESULT?

When we compare this diet with many other diets out there it's easy to see that the Ketogenic diet allows you to consume foods that contain a wide range of nutrients, especially when you are using a derivative Carb Cycling. This is primarily because this diet is not as restrictive as some. You can still eat many of your favorite foods and your favorite fruits and vegetables too. While you may end up consuming more fat than you're typically used to, you'll be consuming different types of fat. This means you'll burn those fats throughout the day so you won't have to worry about gaining weight.

When you start the Ketogenic Diet you won't be eating a lot of bad fats, salt or sugar. As long as you stick to the diet and you eat sensibly there's no reason why you should not lose weight.

For those that need the variety that carb cycling does, it may be a viable alternative. The key is if you are able to truly eat low carb on the days you are supposed to.   If more discipline is needed, carb cycling may be a better approach after you have obtained goal weight and want to ease back into the world of carbs.

Evelyn Carmichael

CHAPTER 7. REFERENCES

1. Dashti HM, Mathew TC, Hussein T, et al. Long-term effects of a ketogenic diet in obese patients. *Exp Clin Cardiol*. 2004;9(3):200-5.

2. Gupta L, Khandelwal D, Kalra S, Gupta P, Dutta D, Aggarwal S. Ketogenic diet in endocrine disorders: Current perspectives. *J Postgrad Med*. 2017;63(4):242-251.

3. Howarth KR, Phillips SM, MacDonald MJ, Richards D, Moreau NA, Gibala MJ. Effect of glycogen availability on human skeletal muscle protein turnover during exercise and recovery. J Appl Physiol (1985). 2010 Aug;109(2):431-8. doi: 10.1152/japplphysiol.00108.2009. Epub 2010 May 20. PubMed PMID: 20489032.

4. Samaha FF, Iqbal N, Seshadri P, Chicano KL, Daily DA, McGrory J, Williams T, Williams M, Gracely EJ, Stern L. A low-carbohydrate as compared with a low-fat diet in severe obesity. N Engl J Med. 2003 May 22;348(21):2074-81. PubMed PMID:

5. Volek J, Sharman M, Gómez A, et al. Comparison of energy-restricted very low-carbohydrate and low-fat diets on weight loss and body composition in overweight men and women. *Nutr Metab (Lond)*. 2004;1(1):13.

Published 2004 Nov 8. doi:10.1186/1743-7075-1-13

6. Yancy WS Jr, Olsen MK, Guyton JR, Bakst RP, Westman EC. A low-carbohydrate ketogenic diet versus a low-fat diet to treat obesity and hyperlipidemia: a randomized, controlled trial. Ann Intern Med. 2004 May 18;140(10):769-77.
7.

Read on for an excerpt of Evelyn Carmichael's book *The Essential Handbook to Turmeric and Ginger*, **now on Amazon.**

THE ESSENTIAL HANDBOOK TO TURMERIC AND GINGER

THE ANTI-INFLAMMATORY DUO THAT WILL CHANGE YOUR LIFE

By
EVELYN CARMICHAEL

Copyright © 2017

Evelyn Carmichael

INTRODUCTION

Many of us are more than happy to rely on prescribed medication to help us cure a wide variety of ills. But did you know that people all over the world have been using spices to help relieve and even cure a variety of conditions?

Turmeric and ginger are two of the most powerful and commonly used spices that are known to fight inflammation, infections, and so much more.

Even though we in the western world are used to taking prescribed medications, some of us are just starting to discover the real benefits of these ancient yet highly nutritious spices.

Let this book show you the benefits of turmeric and ginger. Discover how you too can use the natural power of these spices to help you feel better and prevent a variety of ailments.

Let this book also show you how to use these ancient spices, and learn how to cook a few delicious meals and treats, that can help you benefit from the way they work.

Evelyn Carmichael

CHAPTER 1. THE HEALTH BENEFITS OF TURMERIC

Turmeric is thought to be one of the healthiest spices you'll come across. This spice, like ginger, contains a wide range of nutrients and compounds, and has incredible anti-inflammatory properties.

Turmeric's origin is from a plant found in southern Asia and India is still the world's largest source of the flavorful spice. In fact, it is the main spice used to make curry. But the root of the turmeric plant is the source of which medicine, food colorings, and even cosmetics can be originated from. With an active compound known as curcumin, this spice really has a lot going for it

Let's take a close look at just some of the health benefits of this wonderful spice:

Anti-inflammatory properties and absorption

Turmeric naturally contains over two dozen anti-inflammatory properties that can help to reduce swelling. Curcumin may well be the most powerful of the bunch, but is hard to get the amount you need and for your body to absorb it in the amounts found in curry recipes. To get the full benefits of the curcumin in Turmeric, it is recommended to use turmeric extract. Furthermore, recent studies have shown that to better absorb the turmeric extract, taking it with black pepper is extremely beneficial. While swallowing a couple of peppercorns may seem strange to you, be aware that some studies show absorption rates increasing to 2000%. Lately, you can find Turmeric (or labeled as curcumin) with black pepper together as an extract in the health food store.

Managing arthritis

Those who suffer from arthritis are frequently in pain, and turmeric can help. Thanks to the active properties found in curcumin, it can be used to help combat the associated pain and discomfort sufferers often feel. Incredibly, those who had taken curcumin as part of a trial were found to have a little less pain, and other symptoms.

Anticoagulant properties

Turmeric is thought to work as an anticoagulant by preventing platelets from sticking together, turmeric prevents blood clots from forming and remaining. This in turn, will help prevent heart attacks and strokes. Please speak to your doctor before you decide to use turmeric as an anticoagulant.

Antidepressant

Incredibly, it's thought that this lovely-tasting spice can work as an antidepressant. When used as part of a study in a laboratory, and on animals who were considered to be depressed, it was found that turmeric helped to relieve some of their symptoms. Furthermore, when this spice was used in human patients, it was thought that it has the same effect as Prozac when it comes to managing depression.

<u>Lowering blood sugar levels</u>

Adding a little bit of turmeric to your diet is thought to help reduce blood sugar levels in those with type 2 diabetes. It's also considered to be effective at helping to reverse some of the side effects that are associated with hyperglycemia, and insulin resistance. Those with type 2 diabetes should consider adding a little turmeric to their diet each day.

<u>Alleviating pain</u>

Turmeric extract is thought to have more anti-inflammatory agents that help relieve pain then many over the counter pain killers. In fact, many people use turmeric extract instead of an aspirin or other painkiller. While you should always take any pain medication that has been prescribed by your doctor, knowing that turmeric can help means you may be in a little less pain very soon.

<u>Lowering cholesterol levels</u>

We all know that the foods we consume can have a direct impact on our cholesterol levels. The good news is that turmeric can help to lower those levels. A study that took

place, whereby individuals with high cholesterol were given turmeric showed that when they consumed turmeric daily, their cholesterol levels reduced slightly. In fact, several studies have shown that not only does turmeric extract reduce "bad" cholesterol, it also reduces the plaque buildup in your arteries which is a significant cause of many heart issues and strokes.
Please note that if your doctor has prescribed you cholesterol-reducing medication, you should still take it.

<u>Gastrointestinal issues</u>

Anyone who suffers from gastrointestinal issues such as Crohn's disease, irritable bowel syndrome, or ulcerative colitis should consider consuming turmeric every day. The curcumin that's found in turmeric is thought to relieve the pain and discomfort experienced in these conditions, as well as acting as an anti-inflammatory. In some individuals who regularly consumed turmeric, it was found that they no longer needed to take the corticosteroids that were prescribed.
Please make sure you continue to take any mediation that your doctor prescribes you, even if you're feeling better.

<u>Liver damage</u>

Studies have shown that increasing your intake of curcumin each day could help to delay cirrhosis. This is all thanks to the anti-inflammatory and antioxidant effect that curcumin has. Those who currently suffer from liver damage should continue taking any mediation that has been prescribed to them by their doctor.

Alzheimer's Disease

Turmeric has also been shown to have positive uses in managing Alzheimer's Disease. Curcumin can speed up the clearance of amyloid protein plaques, reducing and the progression and symptoms of Alzheimer's.

To find out more of the amazing benefits and uses for Turmeric and Ginger, please visit https://www.amazon.com/dp/B01N2B8KBN..

Evelyn Carmichael

ABOUT THE AUTHOR

Evelyn Carmichael

Evelyn was in the world of corporate finance before switching her life path after a successful battle with breast cancer. She is a personal life coach, fitness guru, and healthy lifestyle advocate. She has written over 20 healthy living books including the bestselling book The Essential Handbook to Lectin.

Find out more on Facebook or at https://www.amazon.com/Evelyn-Carmichael/e/B01MQYHZLC

Evelyn Carmichael

OTHER BOOKS BY EVELYN CARMICHAEL

Evelyn is the author of the Essential Handbook Series.

Her titles include the following:

<u>Healthy Diet Plans for Health Issues:</u>

<u>The Essential Handbook to Lectin</u>

<u>The Essential Handbook to a Healthy Gut</u>

<u>The Essential Handbook to the Anti-Inflammation Diet</u>

<u>The Essential Handbook to the High Fiber Diet</u>

<u>The Essential Handbook to Reversing Prediabetes and Diabetes: Meal Plans and Recipes to Reduce Your Blood Sugar Levels and Eliminate Diabetes and Prediabetes</u>

<u>The Essential Handbook to the Alzheimer's Diet</u>

Evelyn Carmichael

The Essential Handbook to Hashimoto's

The Essential Handbook for Choosing the Right Diet: A Guide to the Most Popular Diets and if They are Right for You

Anti-Inflammation and Super Foods:

The Essential Handbook to Avocados: The Superfood that Reduce Inflammation and lowers blood sugar, blood pressure, and your cholesterol

The Essential Handbook to Turmeric and Ginger: The Anti-Inflammatory Duo that will Change your Life

The Essential Handbook to Coconut Oil: Tips, Recipes, and How to use for weight loss and in your daily life

The Essential Handbook to Apple Cider Vinegar: Tips and Recipes for Weight Loss and Improving your Health, Beauty, & Home

The Essential Handbook to Superfood Smoothies

Instant Pot Cookbooks:

Healthy Living:

Evelyn Carmichael

AUTHOR NOTE

If you enjoyed this book, found it useful or otherwise then I'd really appreciate it if you would post a short review on Amazon. I do read all the reviews personally so that I can continually write what people are wanting.

Thanks for your support!